Almost Everything You Need To Know As A Dental Assistant That Is Not In The TEXTBOOK!

I use the word Almost: Because we never stop learning Plus it keeps Altizermers away.

In this book you will learn how to advance in your Dental career as an assistant and saving a lot of money in your pocket since starting out in any career you will start with the entry level income but, it will increase if you do your best for your Boss and follow the Dental Assistant Creed & Pledge.

To All My Fellow Dental Assistants In the Dental Field We are not just **a Spit Sucker** as We Have Been Refer To By Some Dentist BUT, We are More than that We are the ones in the office that not only provide the right hand or left hand for the dentist but.....

We Are Also The Ones Who:

Clean: In most cases we are the ones who clean the office with *sometimes* getting paid extra for it and sometimes while on the clock. Sometimes we are even ask to clean the Main Suction Trap with a ToothBrush but, They are **DISPOSABLE!**...NOT A GOOD WAY TO SAVE MONEY. EVERYTHING YOU SUCTION UP GOES THERE AND STARTS TO GROW BACTERIA.

<u>PLEASE DON'T CLEAN THEM</u>

Comfort: Provide comfort for others while sitting in the dental chair

Tip: If your not you should be due to it really does help comfort the patient and regardless of culture, ethics, backgrounds OR stataurt which we all know that exsist in Today's world.

RAW & REAL NOTE: We should not be providing comfort to Doctors for any type of advancement and yes I said it Because, it is RAW and REAL out there and I have had my share of issues from it.

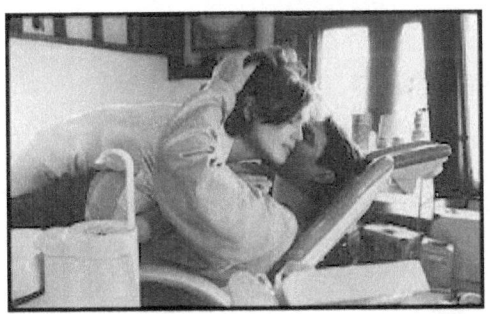

Once had to walk out of a job, I loved so much sobbing and Wife ask why are you leaving...... I just left Because, I was told I would get E.F.D.A school if I slept with The Doctor...WOW , I was **CRUSHED!** and still young ,Learing Life just *excited*

about starting my career in Dental but, Just wanted to share this experience with you incase you ever came across it.

    I feel it is better to know EVERYTHING and sometimes it is better to share an experience it makes another person who doesn't feel good about what they went through to know their are others out there who had to put up with more than tooth decay.

I attach the Creed and Pledge For you Because, It is not always read at School's. I think it should be.

We are loosing that vow to others...

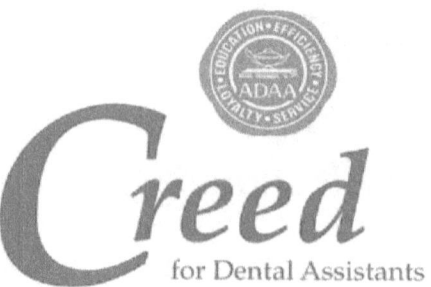

Creed
for Dental Assistants

"To be loyal to my employer, my calling, and myself.

To develop initiative - having the courage to assume responsibility and the imagination to create ideas and develop them.

To be prepared to visualize, take advantage of, and fulfill the opportunities of my calling.

To be a co-worker - creating a spirit of co-operation and friendliness rather than one of fault-finding and criticism.

To be enthusiastic - for therein lies the easiest way to accomplishment.

To be generous, not alone of my name but of my praise and my time.

To be tolerant with my associates, for at times I too make mistakes.

To be friendly, realizing that friendship bestows and receives happiness.

To be respectful of the other person's viewpoint and condition.

To be systematic, believing that system makes for efficiency.

To know the value of time for both my employer and myself.

To safeguard my health, for good health is necessary for the achievement of a successful career.

To be tactful - always doing the right thing at the right time.

To be courteous - for this is the badge of good breeding.

To walk on the sunny side of the street, seeing the beautiful things in life rather than fearing the shadows.

To keep smiling always."

— Juliette A. Southard

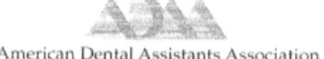

American Dental Assistants Association

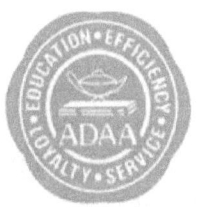

The Dental Assistants Pledge

"I solemnly pledge that,
in the practice of my profession, I will always be loyal
to the welfare of the patients who come under my care,
and to the interest of the practitioner whom I serve.

I will be just and generous to the members of my profession,
aiding them and lending them encouragement to be loyal,
to be just, to be studious.

I hereby pledge to devote my best energies to the service
of humanity in that relationship of Life to which I consecrated
myself when I elected to become a Dental Assistant."

— Dr. C.N. Johnson

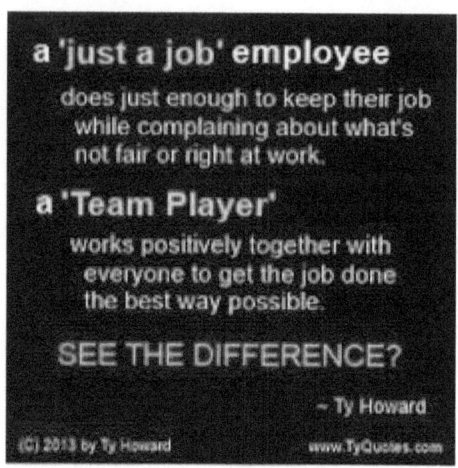

My backgroud: I Took a 2 Year, Free course at a Cleveland Public HighSchool Called Health Careers Center on the East Side, Catching 2 Buses to get to school and wearing white scrubs for 2 years always getting gray at the bottom of my pants in Ohio,Truth be told ...I really wanted the Medical Assistant program but, they were filled up.

    I went ahead and took Dental Assisting thinking maybe ,This is why I use to brush my parent's dentures when I was little.(LOL)Fun Fact about the Author of this book and yes, I had toys, I was just meant to do Assisting and it is amazing how us as Dental Assistants find ourselves in this field and soon it is like second nature like cooking in the kitchen which also, isn't a good thing but will explain that **RAW & REAL** experience later on in this book.

    I also started out in General Dentistry and while in between jobs I saw an ad for an assistant for pediatrics and I thought I don't like other people kids why will I do that (yes young and dumb and all about me at the time) but ,I needed to make money so I applied and realize quickly I can convince kids to open up and get this HUGH X-Ray in their mouth. I eventually ,The Child Whisper at the office.

    I also enjoyed every time a kid would get on Nitrous and tell ALL about their parents or who knows what comes out of mouth of babes right!

    I was offer at that time to work my off days at an Orthodontics office and now that job was awesome it was almost like I was an EFDA after all Because, I did not have to work side by side with a doctor that did or didn't have good chair-side manners and I loved it but, for the record Dr. Arnold D.D.S is a great Orthodontist and the staff was awesome. I will never forget helping kids clean up their face if they came in and look like they came from off the streets and so shy and I would help them and sometimes with the teenagers give them advice if they ask because, I was always going to help someone if needed that is just me but people get that and some truly need someone to listen and as assistants sometimes the dental chair becomes the therapist chair as some of you know it already. I once put braces on a teenager who was all excited and he came from a poor family and he chose his colors and when that weekend came about he drown in Lake Erie and I was impacted by knowing what I placed in his mouth will forever be.......something to think about when you become an EFDA and I hope you do follow the easy way I will show you in this book. Why am I doing this well you might think it is cheesy but I am a christian and I feel if someone would have given me this knowlege my life could have been easier I did not have stable family structure growing up and I learn to make a way in this world by myself which God knew I would use these experiences to help students in my career.

I was also a Dental Assistant Instructor for a few Schools which is why I am writing this because, I know the do's and don'ts and the in's and out's after 30 years.

I would feel selfish if I didn't end my career after 30 years by sharing all this. I want to stop some of these things from happening to you or to comfort you because this career can be hard just like a nurse.

I also worked helping the Army & Marines out which is

great service for our men and woman who serve our country. You will quickly learn our soilders are getting large fillings instead of what they might really need and we all know how large MODLB can turn out in a few years and just image the stress they put on their teeth if they clench or grind which I am sure they do. The Company pays you money also but... DO NOT INTERACT WITH THE SERVICE MEN AND WOMAN OR YOU WILL LOOSE YOUR

CHANCE TO MAKE EXTRA MONEY. IT IS A RULE.

•Career Tip:

Resource Information:

DHMS: Dental Health Management Solutions Contact number is 1-972-763-5639 as of this book being publish is 2018. They pay $130.00 to $150.00 Depending on the jobs which are easy to do. Most the time it is a half a day. They also pay for travel and reimbursement if you would like to take it to the next level. Like with anything it is what you put into it.

ADAAA: Become a member to the american dental assisting association

C.E: Can be found on www.crest.com

Jobs: www.dentalpost.net = fill out completely

Remote Area Medical Corporation (R.A.M): Contact information https://www.ramusa.org If your needing experience or to reach out to help your community plus it is a great way to meet others in the dental field which is" a small world after all " as you may or may not know yet in your career. Please be mindful of that for you never know when you will run into a former co-worker or employer or need to use them for a reference remember everyone needs help at times and these people who wait in line for hours on end just to get a tooth extracted for free they are needing comfort also or a sincere smile. Don't just do it for show do it from the heart. I have done it a few times in my career and it is rewarding knowing you help others.

Assistant Tip:

- Vaseline it is cheap and it shows you care , Lube up those lips and especially the corners so they won't wake up the next day with crack corner lips.

- Offer a bite block:It helps the patient jaw especially if they already have TMJ.

- If using a Rubber Dam : Trim by the nose so it

doesn't bother them , it is bad enough having people in your personel zone.

- Try not to talk over the patient about personel stuff with the doctor or anyone in the room helping especially if it has nothing to do or patient is not included in the conversation.

I also was an Office Manager and some patients would call me and tell me why they where leaving the practice that would be one of many some was to rough.

They are their for your time and talent because Dental is an Art!

AND....

If you don't think you have talent it will come....Have patient with yourself.

- When bibing a patient fold it at the top and you do it for 2 reasons: #1 so it doesn't rub the patient neck & some have Thyroid issues and #2 is it keeps it from ripping on the top from the bib chains which should be wiped after each patient otherwise, it is like taking a necklace off a stranger and putting it on you and all that sweat. You see where I am going because, it could be your Mama in that chair next time and don't clean extra just because, She is your Mama. (Joking in a way) .

I also have had expierence in the Big City life taking the Subway or some call it the Rappit and wearing the cute little outfits Downtown and then going shopping afterwards or walking all the way home for exercise in my good old days that or I had no money at times because, one income and being an assistant...It has provided for me being a single mom to a wife who husband didn't have work or one used me because, I had a job and why am I sharing this because, it's time to have another RAW & REAL FACT! This goes for man or woman assistant but people see you in scrubs they see JOB and that is an attractive part for some so becareful with that also.

    I really do hope whoever buys this book really takes in everything and helps you be the Best Assistant you can be and I mean you worry about you and help others at the same time to often we get burn out yes Doctor , yes Front Office, Yes Hygiene. Helping everyone on the team and sometimes not all the time. It is not return and you get unnotice and put up with stuff behind the scenes just keep your chin up because, It always pays off as long as you don't give up and throw in your spit sucker.

Doctors need good Assistants these days, We can not allowed this profession to loose what we work so hard for because, of a few hickups or bad apples in the field. I am seeing so much go on these days behind the scenes in different offices that we have to try to fix and move on and with that being said before, I go any further with how to advance I would like to address a few things before hand so I know I am not only trying to help you advance but also help the office as a hold.

    Doctors are tired of Gossip in an office (Really should go to work to work if you make a friend along the way that is great but your job is your bread and butter and less gossip better you are with keeping your job. The treatment rooms are paper thin keep that in mind if your new.

Watch what you say! Here is a good one to talk about I never thought I would hear someone talk about having a yeast infection in front of their patient like REALLY? I could not believe I heard that because, Where is the patient head when your working. Example of what we need to watch what we say.

P.P.E - It is becoming a dangerous world out there when it comes to germs so please if you are slacking because of years in the field please protect yourself with all these harsh chemicals that we use to kill some strong fighting dieseases. If your a student right now pay attention you will have many exams that will go over infection control. **Treat everyone as if they have something because we are living in a time of great deception.**

Neck Issues: Exercise from a physical therapist- sit straight up look to your right shoulder with head parrell with shoulders then tilt head down to look at armpit and wait 5 seconds repeat for each side a few times it really does help.

Cramp Hands: Stretch those fingers throught out the day

Peroxide: Removes blood also great oral rinse

Publix's Stores: They offer free RX so if you can't afford because of no insurance or for your patients.

Doctor: Lay their gloves for them , Offer them a cup a coffee, They sign your paycheck and gave you a job , you should be working at all times, something always needs done and they see who is working hard even when their our no patients at the time, everyone has slow times.

Waiver verses Vaccanations: Your employer is REQUIRE by law to offer you the hepatitis B vaccine and if you don't know this for those who have had it at the start of their career needs to after 10 years have your blood check to make sure your still protected and if not then get another one for a booster. Tetinus shot is require because you will get poke and if old at least your going to be protected. There is only one you! if not sign the waiver for the office.

C.E - Continue education you must comply with your state and the National Dental board. I like to keep mine in order and in a binder with year on each folder in the binder. They do audit and some schools do not let you know this and you need to start early so your not trying to get all these c.e last minute same with your chemical dependcy and CPR.

C.P.R- so important to have let me give you a real life expeirnence when I was working on a child a boy age 11 and he was in the papoose board which is very important to use when a child would not lay still but we will discuss that next but going on I was the head holder to protect him from moving and getting hurt and this not an easy job and my back is messed up from it till this day but it was my job at the time and I was going to protect him. I heard the boy grasphing and I look up at the Doctor and E.F.D.A and said he is choking and they just sat there and did nothing next thing I know I got up and ripped him out of the papoose and he was a few inches shorter than me , yes I am a shorty, anyways I first wanted to slap him on the back when all of a sudden i rememenber C.P.R class and knew I should do the hymlick instead. He had his hands arouund his neck saying I am dying and I said not today your not! On the 3rd attempt the Stainless steel crown aka s.s crn shot out and hit the wall Bing, Pong, Bing! it went! The office manager came down and told the parents but the office did not follow protocol which was should have called ambulance right away.

I can not wait to get into how to become an EFDA and how easy it can be to change the Dental Assisting world for the better.

R.D.A Verses C.D.A- R.D.A is a register dental assistant and each state qualifications are different some you don't even have to take a Dental Assisting program if the doctor is willing to train you but here is the thing about just applying for your R.D.A you won't know anything and you really do need to be train so you can apply for your C.D.A which is Nationally Certified and that is important because, your not only bettering yourself but you are showing anyone in the dental world you are serious making this a long career because, it can be to many are quitting but it can be a long career for you if you take proper care of your health and posture! Very important.

    Taking your C.D.A is an exam through Dental Assisting National Board and they are awesome they help you keep track of your C.E's , give you chances for Scholarships, Contest for money if your number is pick that month. It is a community for Dental Assistants and to be part of it you must take the exam which I studied morning , noon and night because it is a 300 dollar exam give or take depending on when you purchased this book.

    They have different exams for you and the more you add to your RDA or CDA the more you can do for your Team at your office. You use to have to wait to take the CDA but now they have the N.E.L.D.A exam which is National Entry Level Dental Assistant. Once you achieve this you can move on to your EFDA exam and so on.

    Everytime you test you are one step closer to success and some doctors might reimburse you for the test or maybe since the cost is so much less by not doing it yourself more doctors would be on board and paying for it and ...

If any Doctor is reading this, You should because, It will help you and more time you have the more patients = More accounts receivable= more $ which should be shared with your team because, it is hard working on the salary we have and some dotors don't offer bonuses at all.

To learn but some parts of it you must practice! I know the fee's can be high and can cost up to if not more 17,000 if you go though a program that teaches

Administrative or Chairside now I am not saying it is not a great program because all your work is done for you but I have to have a wow factor here soon and you might be floored to find this out and maybe a little late but that is ok because you understand why I am writing this book and maybe you can gain something else from it.

So here I was with great students and I mean to tell you, I have had all kinds of students some I thought would never get a job as Dental Assistant because of things I mention earlier to be honest I never met a man as an assistant until I started teaching men who where getting back into the workforce and in some big cities there are male assistants and doctors do enjoy it because, Some have even gone golfing with their employer and why not if two men can work on a car together why not chairside.

    I truly feel we should have more male assistants in the field. I once taught someone who couldn't read and write much at all but she made it with lots of TLC and going over it again and again , that is how some learn. Sharing this incase you are ever a Dental Instructor yourself.

    Most who sign up for Dental Assisting are wanting a better life so you must help those who are less fortunate including helping them finish the course don't be a cold Instructor and say your teaching them if your heart is not in it.

To be honest at the office and the time in School is different than work and some are working trying to make it and some are even doing things they should not be doing just to make it and I can't live with that so I give my all as an Instuctor so they can make it but I get so frustrated when others don't help others out and Doctors won't give them a chance.

    What I have to say to you is Keep trying don't give up and apply again and again and sometimes the ones who hire often are the ones who are hard to work for but you have to get your foot in the door.

I appreciate Dr. Hudec D.D.S and His brother for giving me My Chance, My Foot in the door, and I appreciate HoughNorway Dental office for letting me do my externiship there on the East of Cleveland.

It is where I am from have to give a shout out!

One of my favorite schools of all time was CIDMA (Cleveland Instuite of Dental and Medical Assisting) I wish they were all over but they are only in Ohio, Because they taught me how to be an Instructor and they still gave me a chance to teach with no experience and time to get my CDA and encourage me to do so, I love to give a shout out to them but also so others know that the school really cares for their students. They also give you everything to get started in your career without loosing an arm and leg.

    It was funny starting there the students bet I would only make it 2 weeks but I make it 3 years and would still be there if I didn't marry and move away. Why was there a bet ? Because to be RAW AND REAL it was an inner city school with some getting a second chance.

When you Know you show others you care really care about them bettering themeselves well then you can not go wrong as an Instructor if you ever become one, which you can do it and if you do always give your all to them because you are the first to impression for them in the Dental world. The funny thing is the person I replaced was someone I had a conflict with and oh most got into a fight with at a past job we work at and yes I said and she had a close relationship with the doctor and she was very protected over the doctor.

I had issues with our employer who was drinking on the job and this wasn't the first boss I encounter with that issue because, it is out there.

I was going to have to stand up for the patients because they were just kids she was working on and yes it is not an easy job even for doctors at times and dealing with home life not that it is when you need to get help or take a break which is what I have had to do from time to time in my career because, it can be nerve wracking dealing with difficult patients or staff members themselves and I hate to say this but you will see if you haven't already some people can try to do things to get you to leave the office, If it a family work enviorment and sometimes it is better to just leave but before you do always have another job to keep providing for your family.

    I have had times I just couldn't stand another minute there. I have walk out of places doctors throw things or other assistants I have watch first hand take pictures of another assistant work with cell phone and run upstairs to tell on them but to find out they were not being honable in their profession than the person who was trying to work but missed it which in that case always double check your treatment area and hoses always she make sure no splatter blood is left on treatment room lights or hoses which are missed places and while we are here also make sure you make sure the footrest is clean and reostadt can get dirty after alwhile.

    Getting off track but getting back to the Radiology issue here I had students saying no one will give a chance all because they did not have it so what I found out is you don't need to sit for the course don't need to take it but !!!! you don't have to if you can truly study on your own and go to DANB website and fill out the application and you will go to the Pearson location near you and take exam but there are a few issues with that and that is if you don't learn in a school setting then your not getting everything you need but you can self teach and if possible practice placing the rinn-kit in a co-workers mouth or at the school if they will let you but that is one **WOW FACTOR** by pass the course get the book to study Radiology and practice test off DANB website which you can find on my resource page I made up to be a place you can find your everyday items just, save it on your desktop. https://dentalindex.weebly.com and now getting back to Radiology, take the test and better study for it but once you have that you need:

Nitrous next, Sealant and Coronal Polishing

Once you have all these then move on to studying for your EFDA exam buy a book off EBAY, Like I did for 20 bucks I got mine from Ohio state used books or look at a second hand book store to study for it, then talk to your boss if he is wanting you to be an EFDA (and sadly most don't pay for the course) but ask if they will show you the hands on part of putting fillings in who else can teach you better or watch on YouTube and so on and you study the exam material ,So instead of paying 4,000 if not more for school which we as assisants can not afford to begin with especially when some bosses promises things like bonuses but never provide them ,sorry to say it is out there and if your bless stay where your at the grass isn't always greener on the other side.

    I understand some people will be upset with me sharing this knowledge but if they needed this information I would be glad to help them. It is the right thing to do and too big of a secret to keep it to myself and I say secret because anyone could call and ask them do you need to sit for the course or just take the exam and some assistants have done this for so long they can do it , I know they can!!! if that is you , I totally understand if you put this book down for a minute and print your application out online for your exam but be ready first you only have so many days to sit for exam. *BE PREPARED*!

    Please remember earlier about the

teenager who passed away what you put in someones mouth could really last a lifetime, Take pride in your work, and whatever you do DON'T CUT CORNERS! Now that I just saved you 1,000's of dollars your small investment in my book was worth it if you do it for yourself! The exam can be found on once again the DANB direct website is www.danb.org and email: danbmail@danb.org , CRFDA and theses are the catorgories you will need to test in:

- Anatomy, Morphology and Physiology (AMP)

- Impressions (IM)

- Temporaries (TMP)

- Isolation (IS)

- Sealants (SE)

- Restorative Functions (RF)

- There is no longer a Placing Topical part of the exam as of this year 2018

<u>Here are DANB Pathway requirements for the application:</u>

Pathway I - Current or former CDA cerificant whose certification lapsed no more that two years ago. Must have your License number (

Reminder / Binder is great!)

Pathway II-Graduate of a commission on Dental Accrediatation (CODA) Accredited dental assisting or hygience program or Registered Dental Hygienist (RDA) . Yes you are reading correclty Hygienst can do fillings also if they took this exam. How much better would the dental world be if the doctor is not burn out from leaning over all day when it would help our neck and back out if we were to switch from our Dental Chair Perch to the drivers seat and finish up the work. Yes doctors make a lot of money but they have bills also more than we do and stress of running the whole office and trusting in their staff to do right even when the cat is gone the mice should work. The doctors in this field have the highest suicide rate and we can help that if they help us in return, some doctors are great doctors and some are not some are better with their employers and some are not. I feel a great assistant can help their Doctor ease their stress and know they have their back. I once had that but the doctor still new and admitted they don't teach doctors the business part of it just like we don't get taught everything in school but we are expected to know. This business could be so much better if we all realize how important each part of the team is and yes team there is no(I) in team.

    No office queen madonna please , spread the work load, I use to stand in my classroom doorway and put my arms out and said no one is leaving till everyone cleans us a happy lab is a clean lab and here we had all grown ups men and woman of different backgrounds singing Barney Clean Up Song , Students started it for the record but it was fun and educational all in the same moment. I made sure each student knew what they were doing before they left and that is at any school I taught at.

I am sharing this because, I wanted you to know my background.

Pathway III- Employer work experience and EFDA or Restorative Course/program

WOW.... if I had only known this all these years!

Take a minute let it sink in that you can do it now if your already CDA!!!!!!!!! YAE

Well now you do :) the information is right there for you but who really breaks it down. The job market is floaded with assistants so I wouldn't put it off to long. Maybe this will help increase our wages and help take the load off the doctors. If this could get better for everyone on the team and patients because they will see the less stress out staff.

I had a chance to do a bucket list and interview for a hospital job for the state and they don't have it any better than a private practice. I see issues everywhere and so much behind the scenes that patients don't see.

 I hate to say this but the industy is floaded with so many addicted people to Achole or drugs.

Why do we have to take a yearly dependcy course ?

Why do they help out doctors and others who are addicts because, it is a stressful job from top to bottom.

So please be caution. ....

Lets go over some of the things on the exam you might be getting nervous about , I know you can do this but here it is most it you already know if your a CDA , you know about tolfirmires and mylar strips and rubber dams well thats a lot already and you know about impressions.

Dental Assistant Tip: if your patient is gagging have them hold one leg up and remind them to breath through their nose and if that don't work tell them to say ha haaa ha a few times it clears the back of their throat and sets it up faster. If your patient starts to get sick , I hope your teammates would help you because I have seen first hand needing help and someone walks right by. Don't be that assistant.

Resources: Dental apps on playstore to practice

Pronounce app: for hard words when studying and all languages

Cross Cantamination: I have seen first hand someone grabbing the office phone with Gloves on ....NO! Patients see that in waiting room and plus it is gross they don't know if clean or dirty. Don't bring file up to Front office with gloves on they are not require to have the Hep B vaccine like we are. Don't go in drawers to get something with dirty gloves on use cotton pliers. When extracting teeth keep extra water in a patients cup to rinse lines incase tooth debrie gets caught up in surgical suctions. Don't scratch your bottom or men you know lol,I have seen that also.

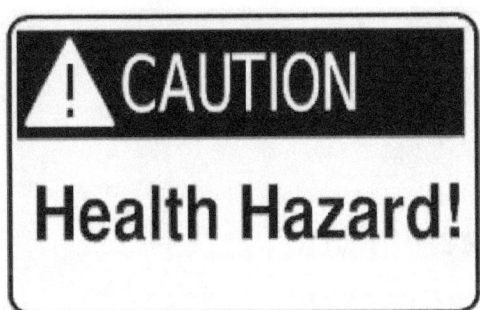

Order things off my site if you need to practice for EFDA or even Orthodontics and so much more, it is there to help you.

Honesty: If you make a mistake own up to it and when something big happens your employer knows you always told the truth.

How in the Heck do we Remember which teeth are which?

Counting Teeth: If you start on the right and finish on the right you be right! and remember these numbers and you can't go wrong unless you forget to count the missing tooth that they may not have had or lost. #1,#16,#17,#32 ,#8,#9,#24,#25 remember those and count forward or back.

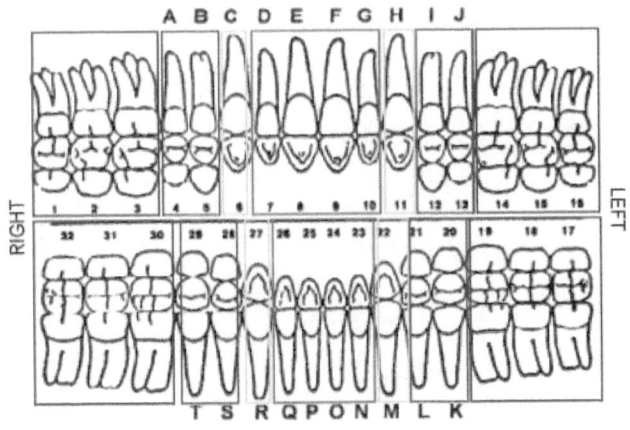

When In The Drivers Seat: Sitting in The Dentist chair that the DDS operates from , you now have time to work without the boss right there but while doing so keep in mind you must stay on schedule while talking and working can be great it can be a distraction, Just a tip and plus now your back and neck can have a break! Just ask the patient to list his or her neck up don't be shy! Protect your body, you only have one and you will be no good later on in the years ......TRUST ME.

3-Position and postures:

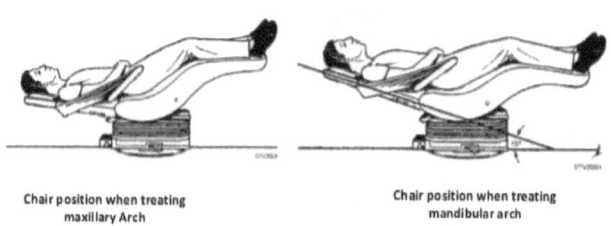

Chair position when treating maxillary Arch

Chair position when treating mandibular arch

Crowns: If trying crowns on put a 2x2 gauze open up and lay it in back of mouth to keep it from dropping

Tip: Can use Composites to fix Temporaries also to match shade of your patient (Even over a differenet material or Brand).

Example: #8 Shade is D2, Temp. material is Shade A2, Just layer it and cure, also to match shade of your patient and Dental Assisting Schools Most don't teach it but, We still have to do it, So watch videos, if never done.

Rubber Dam Clamps: Place floss on it to keep it from falling in throat.

Little Tips (For those that don't know):

1<u>Temporay Crowns</u>: Make sure you check contacts first with floss, don't leave gaps between teeth it will make the seat appointment harder, Make sure Bite is ok most importantly before the patient leaves and one trick is to have them bite down on a piece of shim stock or articulating paper on the opposite side and with temp in place and if paper slides out they are hitting to high and only adjust the blue marking once patient bites up and down and side to side. (

Sometimes you have to show them by taking your mask down or I like to use my hand and rub my fingers side to side or up and down) to help the patient and doctor out. If the contacts are two tight....What to do is take a small piece of the articulating paer and place it in a locking divice of hemostadts and place interproximally (inbetween) the teeth and place temp or permanent crown for that matter same way and tug on paper then pull crown off and if marking , that is your culprit! Always make sure it is shinny , get up and take it to the lab using the lathe and water with course and fine if you can course first then polish it will look prettier even if off some. Can make anything pretty today add a little shine to it.

2**Safety Note:** Really should not wear gloves with lathe wheel,I once was told an assistant broke all her fingers by doing it with gloves on plus if no shield is on it then it splatters if no safety glasses, so please protect eyes from those tiny grains no matter how tired you are and want to cut corners, not on you , never on you or public health, Seen it to often! I am sorry I am not surgar coating it but, we don't care much for sugar anyways in this feild. Unless it's the holidays. I will miss the free cookies!

3Sometimes patients don't need Root Canals , I have been taught the nerve can bruise itself and if no infection I would get a second look. (How Honest of a Person are you working for determines how well you sleep at night!) I have seen it.

4 Send home with your patient a temporary packet made up of a small sterilization bag, 1 2x2 guaze, microbrush and one sheet of mixing pad with a packet of temp. cement and type up instructions, it cuts down on the recementing appointments and they need to keep that crown on.

5 One of doctors pep peeves. When taking impressions and it gets stuck break the two seals with your index fingers by lifting up or down on impression tray with out banging into opposing

arch. In Ortho make sure you get all the clip wires you cut off with the distal end cutters and no they don't go over Ortho either so shadow an office. Also make sure you spray air and water on doctors mirrors you are their windshield wipers. When placing sealants if allowed try using a CTA , Cotton tip applicator it keeps the bite from being high incase you apply to much. Etch and other squeezable items make sure you squeeze first before handing over because it could squirt out and into the patient or their eyes and if not offering glasses to protect their eyes you should be and a blanket!!! We are hot from working patients are cold. Going back to temp crowns or seating crowns use a thin small piece of articulating paper to check where it keeps hitting.

Programs:

Eaglesoft , Soft dent, Dentix and many others can be found on my site at https://dentalindexjr.weebly.com one day it will be just .com but for now type it in this way and they all have tutorials

Clean and water plants

I once went to an office all the plants where dead ...does not look good. He hired a front office person right off the street and she dress like it also , be professional.

Reminder: Don't ever look at the blue light , may not hurt you today but one day like staying in the room during an x-ray!

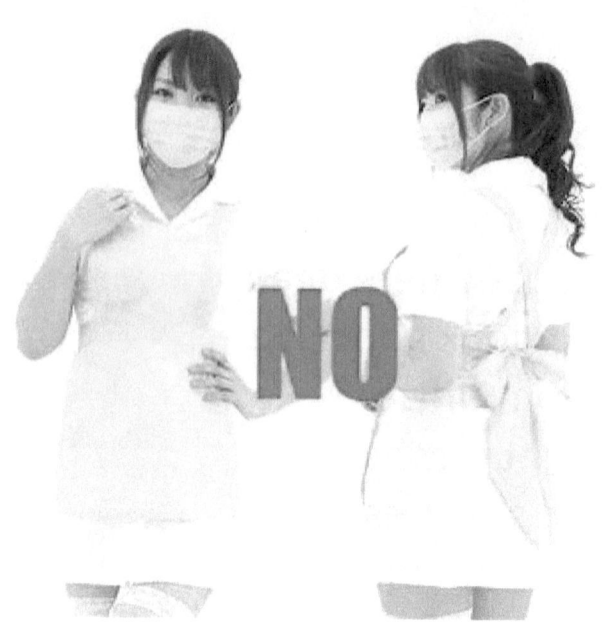

Uniforms: Goodwill if you have to when starting out or stores like Gabes or even the dollar store sells uniforms. I have had more uniforms than regular outfits because it is important to look the part. We are working in people mouths and ladies cover up the TATA's you don't need to show everything and some scrub shirts can show to much. Don't wear thongs if your top is to short , I had a student once bent over to clean and all I saw was thongs. If you wear nails please know with increase in germs , those pretty nails might be putting your life at risk. I know people slack off washing hands and using the new method of hand creams but just had to share we once as a class use glow in the dark powder to see all the germs on our hands after we washed them a few times. I think every school should do that. Scary. ...Good reason not to keep your drinks in the treatment room even if in a cabinet , seen that before because germs do go flying. We tend to get relax in what we do and need reminding, I know I have needed it from time to time. Don't beat yourself up no one is perfect. Learn from your mistakes and move forward. Stay honest and true . Don't set other assistants up ever. Don't hate on one another because your afraid of loosing your job , it is not the new persons fault it is your inscurtitys and that is not coming from the lord so embrace the new person let them feel welcome and most of all Be a Dental Assistant with integurity. What others don't see the lord does. I hope this has helped you in any way shape or form , my personel stories, my ways of getting the job done right or most of all the relief knowing you can go ahead and advance yourself without having to pay so much.

Keep everything from each office you work at you never know if you will need that for something later on right down to P.O instructions. You never know where your career will take you and by me always helping the front out that's how I learn to be front office manager by doing that , you can be an Assistant to an office manager by just working in this field I am living proof of it without all this great knowledge , I wish I had.

Reference: Always get a reference letter from employer saves on them getting calls and you know what is being said and put in your career folder so when on interviews you can hand them everything they need right there from Resume, references, Certificates and so on I have them all.

If hot flashes for us older assistants love the new look of headbands , they work great that or its sweat in their mouth!

Never wear tight gloves they cause carpule tunnel if to tight but if two loose can grasp watch when crowns are being cut off catch every little piece should be accounted for or could cut lungs even porclain.

Disposables: Don't reuse impression trays that are

plastic they are disposable unless made to be autoclave same with HVE suctions, see that also!

Be prepared and always one step ahead of the game as I said it . Pre make-up your bags and sterilize the gauze for the patient to take home.

Make sure MSDA now days it is called SDS book is updated for OSHA and your state. Have signatures on the pages in front of book of the training manual should also have yearly stericycle review www.mystericycle.com

Change suction traps often and run the lines each night don't get lazy with it, I have seen some nasty traps after others.

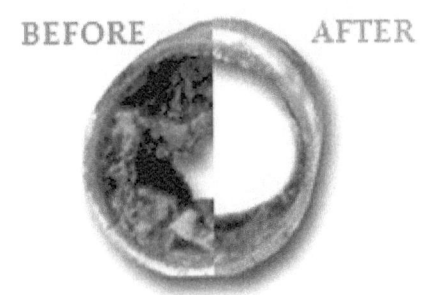

Never use but a microfiber on your treatment room light keeps it from scratching and never use a fabric sheet when washing those they don't work the same.

Different Ordering companys give great deals one I like go to this site https://dds-n-more.myshopify.com?rfsn=2035654.8517e2 target=_blank target=_blank by typing this in you will save.

Your office sales rep can hook you up with discounted toothbrushes that are electronic don't be scared to ask. We have to have nice smiles if this is what we do for a living. I know some doctors don't just do work for free even if I feel and I am sure you do agree that we should get it for free and our family we do so much for the office. I sit here as I write this with number 8 and 9 having MILF composites that our not the right shade and my floss catches it because I was the assistant and it was hard for my boss at the time to do it himself. So please take care of your smiles and expect your employer to treat you as a paying patient and don't go not say anything.

I continue teaching Dental Assisting and I offer tutoring services via the Web just sign up on my site.

I look forward to seeing on DANB website all the new EFDAs !

I leave you with this ...Knock knock...who is there...HIPPA...HIPPA Who....Its HIPPA...I can't tell ya!!!

What does a waitress and a dental assistant have in common? They both ask you how you doing with your mouth full.

Good Luck and eat the night before your test and something in morning so you don't loose contertratrion.

Your fellow Dental Assistant

Theresa Biggs R.D.A, C.D.A

Thank you for your purchase of this book and feel free to subscribe to the website I mention and let me know feedback on this book maybe I will write another.

Dedications:

I would like to dedicate it to my Loving and awesome God and to my amazing Husband Skip and all my Children.

I would like to close with Thanking Everyone in my career for anything you have ever taught me or help as a friend.

I Never will forget each person I worked so closly with and will forever hold a special place in my heart.

From Bosses to the floater in the office.

These Dates are Important and some do not know they exsist!

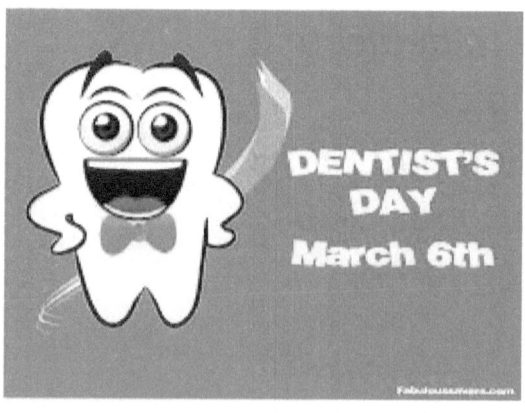

Celebrate
DENTAL ASSISTANT RECOGNITION WEEK
March 4-10, 2018

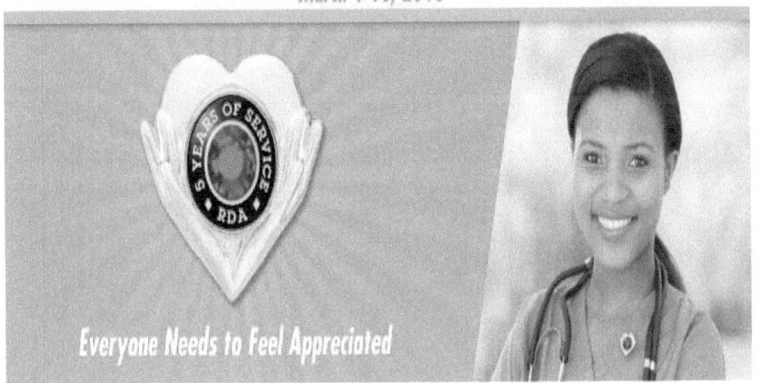

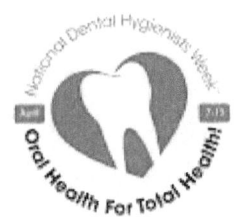
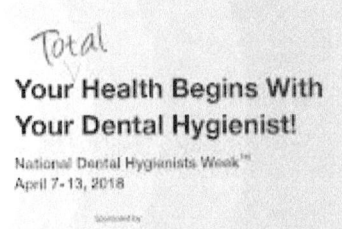

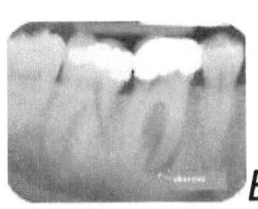 *Example of a Fistula*

www.ingramcontent.com/pod-product-compliance
Lightning Source LLC
Chambersburg PA
CBHW020558220526
45463CB00006B/2363